A CHILD'S JOURNEY THROUGH SEXUAL ABUSE

A Journey of Healing Through Confronting and Exposing Sexual Abuse From Childhood to Adulthood

Cherry Marie

Copyright © 2013 by Cherry Marie
Los Angeles, California
All rights reserved
Printed and Bound in the United States of America

Published and Distributed by:
Professional Publishing House
1425 W. Manchester Ave. Ste B
Los Angeles, California 90047
www.professionalpublishinghouse.com
323-750-3592
Drrosie@aol.com

Cover design : Jay De Vance, III
First printing : January 2013
978-0-9853259-8-5
10987654321

No part of this book may be reproduced, stored in a retrieval system or transmitted in any form or by any means without the prior written permission of the publisher—except by a reviewer who may quote brief passages in a review to be printed in a newspaper, magazine or journal.

For inquiries: mscherry007@gmail.com

Dedication

To all who were abused and never survived to tell their stories:

Even though your lives were cut short by horrible abuses inflicted upon you, your lives and sufferings were not in vain. Even though you left loved ones behind who hurt and grieve for you, I know, as you know, your spirit is at peace with God. You have returned to your Creator, who has the final word regarding all things.

To Dr. Maya Angelou:

My caged bird sings, too, and now she is free. Thank you for your courage and truth. You have inspired many to look to the hills from whence cometh their help.

To Ms. Oprah Winfrey:

Thank you for being so real and transparent even though you were attacked for doing it. Thank you for sharing your sufferings with me and the world. We all want a better life, and you have taught us how to achieve it. Selfish is not your name, but love is.

A Very Gracious Thank You

I am always grateful to the Most High God who gave me the breath of life and the talent to write. I am proof that there is a God. This book would not exist if God did not exist. Thank you, God, for healing me, and all who read this book.

Thank you, mother, for always loving, supporting, and encouraging me.

Thank you, Rev. Rick, for helping me to become a better person. I have learned a great deal from your life.

Thank you, Mr. Jimmy De Vance, III, again for providing your excellent artistic services. Thank you for your love as well.

Of course, thank you, Dr. Rosie Milligan, who has been a mentor, a friend and one who is always willing to help anyone.

I am forever grateful to you all.

Love,

Cherry Marie

Table of Contents

Introduction 7
Chapter 1: Where Did It Begin? 9
Chapter 2: Spirit, Soul & Body – Know Thyself 13
Chapter 3: Once Upon A "Me" Time – My Story of
    Sexual Abuse 17
Chapter 4: Unseen Forces At Work Against Us 25
Chapter 5: Your Story 27
Chapter 6: How Ya Feeling? 29
Chapter 7: Forgiving Your Enemies 33
Chapter 8: A Sickness – Not An Excuse 35
Chapter 9: I love Myself 37
Part II: Little Healing Messages 41
    A Child's Trust In You 43
    The Son Of A Drunken Rapist 45
    A Hole In Your Soul 47
    Prayer Changes Things And People 49
    Born To Be Loved By God 51
    The Greatest Love 53

INTRODUCTION

In the Holy Bible, God commanded the man and woman to be "fruitful and multiply" (Genesis 1:28). The act of sex was originally a beautiful expression of love and affection. It was designed to procreate the earth. Since the fall of mankind and institution of rebellion, sex, like everything God created, has been twisted and perverted into something God never intended it to be. Sexual abuse is a perfect example of this.

A Child's Journey Through Sexual Abuse is one of the most important books you will ever read because it confronts and exposes the truth about sexual abuse completely. It is my desire to allow the words written in this book to help bring about healing to any or all who have suffered, including the abusers. We hold the keys to our healing. In order for us to become whole, we need spiritual, physical, and psychological healing. We are all sick or not whole, and we are in need of healing from something.

This is why life is so full of pain because we are causing it. We are all responsible.

Healing always begins with the truth. It is not my truth, not your truth, but God's truth. That is the only truth we need.

So, if you are ready, let's walk down the healing road together. I've got your hand and God's got your back. We can do this! Let the healing begin.

Love, Peace, Joy…

Cherry Marie

CHAPTER 1

Where Did It Begin?

I am a person who loves to discover the origin of something. I love to know how it all got started, how something began or was created. Origins provide a starting point for something. Everyone and everything has an origin. Sexual abuse did not begin with my experience or your experience. It didn't begin with anyone in our lifetime today.

Sexual abuse began as early as during biblical times. That was more than two thousand years ago. The purpose of sexual abuse, than anything, is and was spiritual. Clearly, from a biblical perspective, it has been used as a weapon; an assault against humanity initiated by unseen diabolical forces. The ultimate goal is and was for the destruction of mankind.

Cherry Marie

In the Holy Bible, the book of II Samuel, Chapter 13 clearly provides an example of sexual abuse in King David's family who was the King of Israel at that time. King David had several children. Some of the children were born through different women because King David had many wives and concubines; one of King David's son was Absalom, Absalom had a sister named Tamar. The Bible says that Tamar was lovely. Another son of David, who was Absalom's brother, was named Amnon. Amnon ultimately fell in love or lust with his sister, Tamar, one of King David's daughters. If you read the entire story in Chapter 13, you will see that Amnon used his male friend to entice his sister Tamar to bring him food to his bed. Amnon pretended to be sick. Amnon had made up his mind that he had to have sex with Tamar even though she was his sister and a virgin. After much pleading with Tamar, she brought food into his room and he raped her even though she begged him not to. After Amnon raped his sister, he hated her even more than he lusted after her. Just that quickly, Amnon's guilty conscious made him turn away from his sister whose virginity he stole and changed her life forever. Amnon threw Tamar out of his house by force. He called his servants to do this because he was not able to face her. Tamar became a desolate woman and she went to live with her brother Absalom. The word desolate in *St. Martin's Word English Dictionary* means; empty, uninhibited, deserted, alone, solitary, joyless, without hope, dismal, gloomy, to make somebody feel sad and lonely, make wretched. Surely, anyone who has been sexually abused can identify with how Tamar was feeling.

A Child's Journey Through Sexual Abuse

Absalom eventually ordered his servants to kill his brother, Amnon, after Tamar told him about the rape. I believe there were many other sexual abuse assaults which were not recorded during those and even earlier times. The point is God saw it all. Sexual abuse is a sin committed against God and mankind. King David's family was torn apart because of this sin. Sexual abuse has been prevalent for so long that it is epidemic today. Just as Tamar was left to be alone to live with her abuse, many people in our society have been living desolate as well. It is never good to hold so much pain inside because it will manifest on the outside without your permission. It is like your inner-self is crying out for help even when your outer-self covers your mouth so you don't scream. Drugs, alcohol, pornography, promiscuity, violence of all kinds, obesity, perversions, etc., are all cries for help. God knows you are in need of healing. You don't have to be a desolate woman, man or child. You can recover.

CHAPTER 2

Spirit, Soul & Body
Know Thyself

I realize that many people in this world do not believe they are a created being with a spirit, soul and body. Some people want to believe in a theory that says, "Life came from a big bang or an explosion!" However, theories, including this one, can be easily disproven. Many people, who have walked this earth at some time, eventually realized that God created us all. In the book of Genesis 1:26, we are created in the image and likeness of God. God is a spirit. If you choose to believe a theory over God's own inspired words; that is your free will choice. If you choose to believe God then you must believe that we are spirits, we have souls, and we live in this physical realm in a physical body.

It is important to know thyself if you are trying to heal or recover from anything. Every part of your being is affected when one part of your being is affected. Sexual abuse of any kind affects our spirit, soul and body. Moreover, sexual abuse affects God even more than the person who is being abused. Sexual abuse is a direct attack or assault against our very Creator. Ask yourself, as a parent, how would you feel if your child was abused in any kind of way? Now, multiply that feeling times all the people who ever lived who was abused. Only God could handle all of that pain from knowing that His precious creations were being abused. Yet, it still affects Him greatly. God has an enemy named Satan or the devil. He is a spirit and he hates God and anything God created, especially mankind. God wants the very best for all His creations. The devil wants the very worst for all of God's creations. Sexual abuse, hatred, violence, murder, evil, perversions, theft, abuse of every kind, etc., all come from the devil's influence. It is only because we allow these evils to take place in our lives that they have become so prevalent. It's not God's fault, but mankind's fault for turning away from our true Creator God. We have chosen to live a life without God's influence or guidance. We have opened the door for every evil of every kind to enter in, and we have done this ignorantly. Today, we are still paying the price for "doing it our way," as opposed to God's. Only today, evil is even more vile and prevalent.

A Child's Journey Through Sexual Abuse

We did not invite someone to abuse us sexually, but the person who committed the abuse was not operating or living in God's will. If they were, it would have never happened. They allowed their own spirit, soul, and body to be influenced by their weakness, their past abuse, their twisted thoughts and perversions, which all come from the evil spirit known as the devil (Satan). The old phrase, "The devil made me do it," has some truth to it. Although the devil cannot make us do anything we don't yield ourselves to. Our own free will (in most cases) causes us to do any type of evil.

There have been multitudes of God-loving, God-fearing people in the world who have not only been sexually abused, murdered, mutilated, etc., they were attacked by someone who was influenced by the devil. Someone who didn't realize what they were doing and didn't care. Someone who was psychologically deficient for some reason. There may be many reasons, but they are all under the same plans of God's enemy—the devil.

Fearfully and wonderfully made, we were created in God's image and likeness. We are an awesome creation. Yet, we have drifted so far away from God that only He could recognize us. We are at the bottom of the barrel of all humanity. We have become slaves or robots to a society that has chosen to ignore God and go their own way. God has not forgotten us nor has He given up on us. We must make positive choices in our lives and, collectively, we must make a change. God loves everyone, even the worst person in society. He knows better than we do who is responsible for sexual abuse and any other evil. Yet, we still must choose right from wrong. We can be healed. We can be all that our spirit, soul and body were created to be for God and for each other.

CHAPTER 3

Once Upon A "Me" Time
My Story of Sexual Abuse...

*Sexual abuse has become the "norm" in society because it has een allowed to exist in our homes, our schools, our churches and anywhere else evil exists.

I was born to a beautiful young woman at the age of seventeen ears old. She was already a teenage mom at sixteen. My father as twenty-nine and he had already fathered another child somewhere by someone I never knew. My mother was not able to aise both my sister and me, so to avoid adoption, my father chose to raise me. I never saw my mother again or at least remembered her until many years later. Fathers are created to head the household and protect the family. When all breaking lose all over the country, my father did his best, as a young Black (African American) man in the sixties, trying to raise a baby girl. This is how, at an early age, I knew there was a God. My father always prayed to God on his knees morning and night, "Please God, help me raise Cherry and let me see her graduate." My father showed and expressed love in every way any child could hope for. He was not a rich man in material goods, but he made sure I had food, clothing and a place to lay my head even while his t-shirts had holes in them, which was often. My father worked hard to provide for us. During those years, I do not remember seeing or knowing my mother, but I do remember my father always telling me two things: To never hate my mother and to focus on school, not my looks. That was some of the best advice he ever gave me. I knew my father loved me because he asked God to help him. He used to point out the moon and the stars. While looking up at the sky, he would say, "You see all of that? God made it all!" I believed him. I was blessed to have the experience of many precious memories of my father whom I loved so much.

My father never knew of the sexual abuse that I had to endure throughout my childhood, except one time. One day, my father unexpectedly walked in early from his job around the corner. He found the screen door to our apartment opened. He then, shockingly, saw the teenage neighbor boy on top of his seven-year-old daughter. The boy was trying to rape me, again. He was about twelve or thirteen and he had a young brother who was about nine or ten. They both often attempted to abuse me sexually when no one was around. I was a latchkey kid. My father worked around the corner at a tire company. The neighbors in our apartment building watched out for me most of the time. My father felt that it was safe enough for me to play inside of the apartment complex while he was at work. No one ever expected the Jehovah Witness family had two sons who were molesting little kids.

After my father witnessed that most unbearable horror of me almost being raped by that teenage boy, he looked like he could kill him. He cursed him out of the house as the boy ran next door to his apartment. I was screaming and crying all the time. Then, I went to my room terrified, confused, and ashamed; I felt so bad. I felt worse for my father than myself. I did not even know the word "sex" at that time. I remember kids in the neighborhood referring to something sexual as "the nasty." I was terrified of it. I knew it was bad, but I had no way to prevent it from happening to me. It seemed like I was waiting in my room for hours when my father burst in the room. He then began to unleash his fury, his rage, his disgust, his ignorance all over me with his belt. I just screamed, and yelled, "No, Daddy, no!" He did not stop until his adrenaline was spent. Then he closed my door and disappeared. I heard him talking to someone, but I was in so much pain. I was in pain from that teenage boy forcing me inside my apartment onto the sofa, trying to force himself inside of my body, and that was when my father saved me. He actually did, but why was I being punished? I never got a chance to find out why that boy did that to me. Why he and his brother tried many times behind our building? Why he threatened me again and again if I told anyone? For the rest of my life with my father alive, I believed he carried a shame or guilt from that experience. I can't imagine all that he felt, but it had to be bad because my whelps from the belt took a long time to heal. After that, I felt my father loved me a little less and was shamed. I felt he blamed me for everything and not the teenage boy who was completely responsible for it all. He was even training his younger brother as well. My father died when I was twelve and a half. I loved him greatly and I never held the beating against him. I always felt ashamed because he blamed me and he told other adult people who knew me. It seemed they all looked at me differently after that. When my father died, I had a peace about that particular experience. I was no longer ashamed and I knew that God had told him what really happened was not my fault. I was just a little girl, after all.

That episode of sexual abuse was not my first, nor my last. Ironically, most of all my abuse occurred with two brothers who were always older than I. When I was six years old, my father had a short marriage to a woman who had two sons. One of her sons was thirteen and he was husky. The younger son was ten years old. I was between six and seven years old. My evil stepbrothers verbally and physically abused me when my father and stepmother were not around. The oldest stepbrother threatened me with bodily harm if I told anyone. He used his size to overpower me as well as constant fear. Sometimes they forced me to eat dog food and other in-humane things. I would cry, but I never told. From time to time, the two brothers would jump on top of me, and the bed, and simulate a sex act with our clothes on. They laughed me to scorn because I was powerless. The marriage between their mother and my father ended after a short while. It was a blessing to me. I was no longer going to be their victim ever again. Many years later, I learned that the older brother was addicted to drugs and was in and out of jail. The younger brother had a nervous breakdown and was in a mental hospital. What led to them taking out their evil plan upon my innocent self? I'm not sure, but I do know that something in their earliest childhood contributed to their abuse towards me. Any evil thoughts or plans are encouraged by the devil himself. Even a child is not immune. Most kids do not realize why they are acting abusive. They just act.

One of the most horrific experiences of my childhood involved a female babysitter and her teenage friends. I remember my father had a friend who he often went fishing with. His friend had two small children younger than me. I was about seven or eight. My father was single.

I remember that one day my father allowed his friend's teenage babysitter to take care of the two small children and me. They were between five and six years old. The babysitter was a teenage girl who was very large in size. She had to be fifteen or sixteen, maybe older. She had been the regular babysitter for the two children for a while. Sometime after my father left with his friend, the teenage babysitter went outside and invited her even bigger teenage male friends inside the house where we were.

Cherry Marie

Once inside the house, they all began laughing in the kitchen. We kids wondered what was so funny. We tipped around the corner toward the kitchen and we saw the teenage girl on the floor. We could only see half of her because the wall blocked our view. The teenage boys were taking turns on top of her and they were laughing. We ran back to the room. Before we could close the door, the babysitter grabbed the hand of the small boy and threw him on the bed. He tried to get up, but she held him down. Then she ordered the older girl who was his sister to lie on the bed. They began to cry. The babysitter forced the little boy's body on top of his older sister's body. I just stood in the background terrified. After a while, the kids were laughing with the babysitter. She then took them into the kitchen and told the older bigger teenage boy to sodomize the little girl, but she used another phrase instead of sodomize. The little girl didn't resist, she stood on her feet until he quickly violated her. They laughed at her. Finally, the babysitter wanted me to be initiated. This time I refused. They forgot to make me afraid to refuse. I did not know them, so they never made me feel threatened, at first. After I refused, I walked away from them.

The next thing I knew was that her very big teenage friend was behind me. They took my clothes off and held me while they laughed. Then he began to sodomize me while I cried very loud. It felt like a bowel movement trying to force itself inside my body. Thank God he did not tear my body. He finally let me go. The big teenage boys left the house and the babysitter gave the little kids candy not to tell anyone. She threatened to hit me if I told anyone, but I was already groomed in that area. I never told anyone, especially my father. I had already been previously warned by several other abusers not to tell or else! Something worse was going to happen to me. I remember those little children so well. They had been experiencing that abuse regularly so it became a game, but inside it was killing something within them.

    I had the fortunate experience of hearing another person who had molested me admit it. I was much older and stronger. The abuser was sorry for what he did and I believed him. He changed his life and was a Christian who had completely changed. I was grateful for that experience because at least one person admitted that they were wrong and was a changed person. At the time of my father's passing, he only knew of that one horrible experience of sexual abuse. I am glad that he did not hurt that boy who abused me because he would have probably gone to prison. I would have lost those precious years with him. My father was a good man who did his best to raise me alone. Parents can do all they can do to protect their kids, but evil things may still happen to them. This is the world we have created. In this world, we have allowed the devil's influence and ignored God's commandments. I know the faces and some of the names of those who abused me. I do not hate them. I forgive them. I am grateful to be alive today to be able to help the world heal because God knows we need it.

CHAPTER 4

Unseen Forces At Work Against Us

As I reflect upon my childhood experiences with sexual abuse, I have to add that I have had spiritual experiences in my adult years that directly reflect what happened to me during childhood. People who know the Bible and understand the word of God will understand better when I refer to unseen forces at work against us. Even if you don't understand the word of God, the media is saturated with paranormal movies and reality shows from celebrities who have had some very real experiences with the spirit world. My experience happened when I was asleep. Remember, two brothers much older than me committed most of the sexual abuse I experienced. I was asleep, but I was not dreaming. I was awakened or became aware by two spirits that had no faces. They were two very horrible forms. They were holding me. They felt like prickly thorns sticking me all over as they held me. They were attempting to sodomize me in the spirit while my physical body was asleep. I was very aware as I tried to scream, but my mouth was covered. I could not vocalize the words. I tried hard to scream out, "Jesus!" Finally, it broke forth—the name of Jesus came out loud as I sat up in my room. Just that quickly, I was aware of everything that happened to me and then I saw lightening flash in my room very quickly. It was in the middle of the night and there were no windows in my room. The lightening flashed low so I knew it didn't come from outside. I knew immediately that when I called out to Jesus, He sent his angel to fight in the spirit the demons who were attacking me. After that happened, the demonic spirits left. I cried and wondered why that happened to me. Later, I realized that God allowed me to experience such a horrible thing to make me aware of how real the spirit world is and how it has a great impact upon every human life. Believe it, the devil and his demonic forces are always at work in the spirit behind every evil event in this world. Yet, we are still responsible for the choices we make—good or evil. We are responsible because we all have a free will.

CHAPTER 5

Your Story

It's your turn. Now that you have heard my story, tell your own story. I will leave this chapter open for you to write down your own personal story. Writing down your feelings has tremendous healing power. You may want to share your story with others or keep it between you and God. Someone needs to hear and know your story, so they will be able to heal just like you. So start writing…

CHAPTER 6

How Ya Feeling?

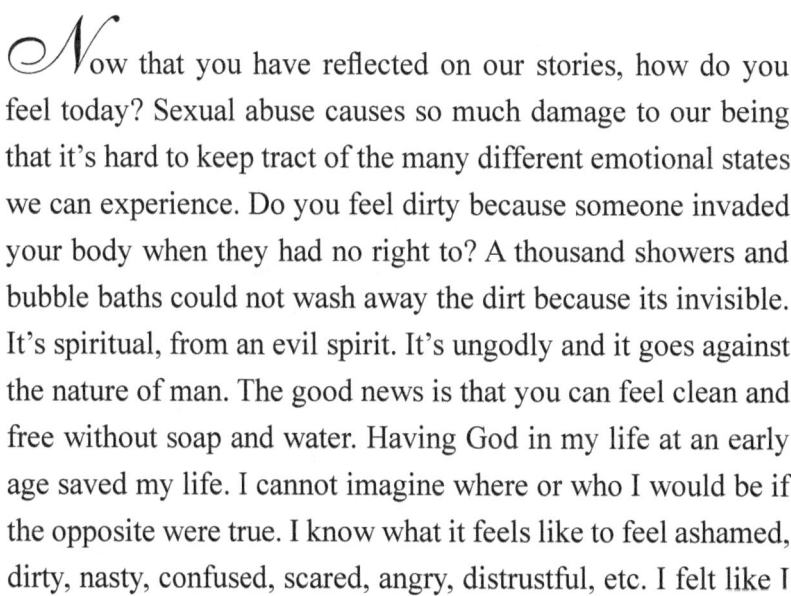

*N*ow that you have reflected on our stories, how do you feel today? Sexual abuse causes so much damage to our being that it's hard to keep tract of the many different emotional states we can experience. Do you feel dirty because someone invaded your body when they had no right to? A thousand showers and bubble baths could not wash away the dirt because its invisible. It's spiritual, from an evil spirit. It's ungodly and it goes against the nature of man. The good news is that you can feel clean and free without soap and water. Having God in my life at an early age saved my life. I cannot imagine where or who I would be if the opposite were true. I know what it feels like to feel ashamed, dirty, nasty, confused, scared, angry, distrustful, etc. I felt like I did something wrong when I took a beating for someone who abused me. Seemingly, we have to carry all of those heavy burdens for the rest of our lives, right? Wrong! It was not our fault. We do not have to carry a single burden. I don't and neither should you.

When I became older, I realized I had to fight for my life because it seemed like someone or something was fighting against me. In later years, I realized how true my feelings would become. I asked God to help me. I wanted to become stronger from within so that no one could ever take advantage of me again. As I grew spiritually, I grew stronger from within. Ultimately, I was free to help others to be free.

Many people have faced deadly experiences involving sexual abuse. Many were raped at gunpoint or with a knife up to their throats. Fear was at the forefront of all of those horrible experiences. Fear was the spiritual and physical weapon used against you. You feared that if you fought back and yelled, you would have been instantly killed. Throughout the history of our world, there have been multitudes that were killed even though they yielded to their abuser. Yet, but for the grace of God, there go I! Thank God, we who have survived have survived to help and to be a blessing to someone else! Those who did not are loved and greatly missed. We do not know why she or he and not me. What we do know is that God has all the answers and He has the master plan. That is all we need to know.

If you do not face your feelings about sexual abuse, you may try to bury them with addictive behavior. You may become addicted to drugs, including prescribed drugs or alcohol. You made bury your feelings in food, gambling, pornography and other sexual abuse. You may be a young person or even an older one who was sexually abused. You may offer your body to other individuals freely because you feel it does not matter anymore. Someone has already violated your right to choose sex. Now you don't feel like caring enough to choose whom you give your body to or how many there will be. It may also be a way of you subconsciously fighting back. You may think you have to be sexually active all the time because someone will try to take it by force anyway. Whatever your weakness is, God is there to help you overcome it. God's enemy, the devil, will always continue to urge you in the wrong direction until you are spiritually, mentally, and physically destroyed. That is the enemy's M.O. for everyone. Believe it or not, throughout history this world has a track record to dispel all of your doubts. Your life is being destroyed by your own addictive behavior because you don't want to face the truth. You will watch and play video games, movies, TV shows and listen to music full of images of demons, the devil, vampires, witches, ghosts, and all kinds of "paranormal" spirits while you won't believe that the devil is real. You are blind.

Anyone who has been sexually abused has the potential to become an abuser of any kind himself or herself. If you don't work through your feelings and the events of your abuse, you may abuse someone who is even close to you. I have now realized that most of, if not all, those kids who abused me were victims themselves. It may not have all been sexual abuse-related, but it was abuse against them. They found a weak little girl who they were able to act out those feelings upon. I know of an older woman who was raped by her two brothers at a very young age. She became promiscuous after that. Later, as a teenage mother, she had several children out of wedlock. She was still a little girl who was devastated by what had happened to her. She held it in many years. No one knew. After her kids were born, she abused them physically and mentally. She did not realize what she was doing. Her children never understood. At some point, she went to a Therapist. She finally talked about it. A lot of damage had already been done, but she was on the road to recovery. She had developed a shopping addiction in addition to her abusive behavior against her kids. It was severe, but she was also working through the many debts she created. God was always there with her and for her. He always wanted to help. When she took the first step, the door opened and she was guided onto the path of healing.

Sexual abuse is like a domino effect, a vicious cycle that will never end until you do something about it. Those of us who are alive who know this truth are in the process of healing. Healing is a process. Like a Christian being "saved." It is a lifetime journey into God's perfection for you. Healing takes time, truth, understanding, forgiveness and a willingness to become better no matter what you feel like right now. Feel better? I knew you would!

CHAPTER 7

Forgiving Your Enemies

$\mathcal{O}$ne of the hardest lessons that I had to learn was to forgive those who wronged me. Some lessons are easier; this one took longer. I felt I had a right to hold on to my feelings against someone who had wronged me. I was wrong. I learned that God forgives me every day when I do wrong because I'm not perfect. I'm still a sinner in the process of being saved. I cannot call myself a Child of God if I do not forgive others when God already has (Matthew 6: 14-15). I have no right not to forgive and neither do you. Yet, you still have a free will choice to choose. Forgiveness is healing to the one who was wronged. You may never see that individual who wronged you again. They will have to answer for their own sin one day. What is right in God's eyes is what matters. The abuse is clearly wrong, but so is the unforgiveness, which is an equal sin, not a lesser one. There is no value, gain or growth in holding a grudge or refusing to forgive anyone at any time for anything. The other person has likely moved on and repented. God has forgiven them and you have not. Are any of us greater than God? We are all going to have to answer to God for the life that we have lived. The best part of healing from sexual abuse is that by forgiving you can be free. You are no longer a prisoner. You are instantly free to move on and out of the prison cell that had you bound by something horrible that happened to you. You are free to move on and out to help save somebody else. The God in you will make it possible for you to be all that you were created to be! All evil in the world can never prevent God from seeing His plans fulfilled.

CHAPTER 8

A Sickness – Not An Excuse

This chapter is especially written for the benefit of all who have ever sexually abused anyone. Benefit? How does someone who stole your virginity, gang raped you, molested your children, raped your grandmother, sodomized your son, etc. deserve any kind of benefit other than torture in hell? We are all sinners in need of salvation. God said, "We have all sinned and come short of the glory of God." (Romans 3:23) We are not here to judge. There are no excuses for this horrible act committed against mankind. People who commit these abusive acts are being punished or tormented already by having committed them. It is an act against God and man's own nature. Even animals know better, which proves that it is unnatural for mankind to do this and therefore a sickness. No person who commits these acts is in their God-given right mind. They may not be insane, but they are sick with a disease like alcoholism, drug addiction, etc. Any abuser can be healed of this sickness. God loves you unconditionally and He is forgiving. You may have been abused yourself, but this isn't an excuse. It is only information to help you on your path to healing. Maybe you don't know why you are doing these things. It is up to you to seek out help through prayer, counseling, and any help you may find. God loves everybody, even you. He can forgive you. You need to ask God for forgiveness and if possible, those you have abused. God has a plan for your life as well. After you overcome your sickness of sexually abusing people, you will have peace. Pray for a personal relationship with God so you can become all that He has created you to be. The devil used you to commit an evil act against another one of God's creations. Your life is not over. As long as you are breathing, God is your healing.

CHAPTER 9

I Love Myself

Have you ever felt that no one loves you? Especially after being sexually used and abused or you have abused others. I love myself. Do you love yourself? If you don't, what is stopping you? If no one in the whole world loved you, would you love yourself? I would because you have to learn to love yourself before you truly love others. How do you do that? First, you must respect life and the Creator of all life that is God. You need to understand how wonderfully He made you in spite of all your short comings, and in spite of all your sins. Next, you need to be grateful for your life no matter how you got here. You are blessed to be alive, so be grateful that God made you special and unique to the world. Learn to appreciate your attributes. You are

Cherry Marie

always beautiful in God's eyes. God has blessed each one of us with talents and gifts to bless the world. There is no reason for you not to love yourself. You are a blessing waiting to happen. Someone needs you. They need your help, your skills, talent and abilities. God needs you to share your love with the world, so you can teach them to love themselves.

SEXUAL ABUSE IS A DISEASE OF EPIDEMIC PROPORTIONS

PART II

Little Healing Messages

1. A Child's Trust In You
2. The Son Of A Drunken Rapist
3. A Hole In Your Soul
4. Prayer Changes Things And People
5. Born To Be Loved, By God
6. The Greatest Love

PART II

A Child's Trust In You

    Trust is something we learn as children. When we get used to the presence of others, we become familiar with them. We come to know them as mother, father, teacher, pastor, friend or other. I was blessed to know my father and I had a very good relationship with him. I trusted him because he never betrayed my trust. He never took advantage of me. Even though I took an unjust beating from him after he walked in on one of my abusers, I never held it against him. He did not know what he was doing. He could have killed that boy, which would have sent him to prison and it would not have changed what had already occurred. My father helped me become the person I am today. Many people have terrible memories of how their fathers, mothers, or others betrayed their trust by sexually taking advantage of them. Some of them allowed others to commit this abuse while they turned away or denied that it ever happened. Never blame a child for something they don't even understand and something they cannot control.

PART II

The Son Of A Drunken Rapist

This is a true story about a child conceived through a vicious rape attack. This story was originally told to a pastor who preached a sermon about it.

There was a woman who was taken at knifepoint and viciously raped. The man who raped her was a known drunk in the community. After suffering through the attack, the woman found that she was pregnant. Only she and God knew how she felt at that moment. The woman ultimately decided against an abortion. Over the course of time, the child, who was the son of a drunken rapist, became a man. A man who became a great preacher who led many people to God.

The point of this true story is that it's not important how any of us got here, But what we do after we get here.

PART II

A Hole In Your Soul

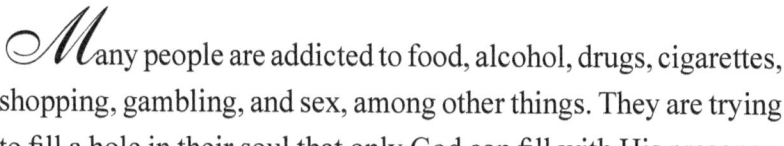

*M*any people are addicted to food, alcohol, drugs, cigarettes, shopping, gambling, and sex, among other things. They are trying to fill a hole in their soul that only God can fill with His presence.

> I gotta hole in my soul
> a hole that won't close
> a hole I feed that never get's full
> a hole where I pour liquor and bull
> a hole I don't see but I smell it with my nose
>
> The hole in my soul is leading me to pimp
> Tempting me with cocaine, heroin and that other hemp

Cherry Marie

The hole in my soul is growing every day
I need a shopping trip to make it through the day
The casino is calling—cha-ching
Cha-ching, can't you hear it?
That hole in my soul get's louder every minute

Oh Lord, please help me out of this predicament
I've tried everything, I'm ready to repent!

PART II

Prayer Changes Things And People

As we consider the epidemic of sexual abuse in the world, we really need help. We need true prayer, not religion. God answers prayers. We need to pray for everyone, including ourselves and our leaders. We need to humble ourselves and ask God to forgive us. We need to ask God to heal our land and heal our people.

PART II

Born To Be Loved By God

Never asked to be born
Never knew what I'd be
But here I am world take a look at me
It wasn't my fault
Someone treated me bad
They took my innocence
And left me so sad
I tried to shake it off
Using different kinds of pills
But nothing made a difference
Until I changed my own will
I called upon God to ask Him to help me

Cherry Marie

He answered my prayers so I'm able to see me
Never asked to be born, but now I'm able to see
God loved me more than Mama and Daddy

PART II

The Greatest Love

This life that we live, with all of its tragedies and enmities, is all about God's love and man learning to love himself and one another. Love is our greatest weapon against our only true enemy, the devil. The greatest love is God's love for us all. Only God can love the most wretched in the world while He loves the sweetest little baby because after all, we were all the sweetest little baby in the beginning. God's love is unconditional. There is nothing that we can do to make Him not love us even when He hates the things that we do. God's love is greater than all the pain of sexual abuse on any kind of abuse. God's love is free even if you refuse to believe for God is love.

www.ingramcontent.com/pod-product-compliance
Lightning Source LLC
Chambersburg PA
CBHW022343040426
42449CB00006B/695